Great Cure and tips about Norovirus outbreak 2023.

Author Dr Dave mosley.

About Norovirus

what is Norovirus:

Norovirus is an extremely infectious

virus that causes vomiting and

diarrhea. People of all ages may become infected and ill with norovirus.

You may develop norovirus disease several times in your life since there are many distinct varieties of noroviruses. Infection with one form of norovirus may not protect you against other types. It is possible to establish immunity to (protection against) particular kinds. But, it is not known precisely how long immunity lasts. This may explain why so many individuals of all ages become ill during norovirus outbreaks. Also, whether you are vulnerable to norovirus infection is also influenced in part by your genes.

Norovirus is also termed the stomach flu or stomach bug. However, norovirus disease is not connected to the flu which is caused by influenza

virus

Content:

Introduction

Human norovirus, formerly known as Norwalk virus, was initially detected in stool specimens collected during an epidemic of gastroenteritis in Norwalk, OH, and was the first viral agent demonstrated to cause

gastroenteritis (1). (1). Illness caused

to this virus was originally identified

in 1929 as "winter vomiting disease"

because to its seasonal inclination

and the frequent majority of patients

with vomiting as a main symptom

Description

Research shows that following a restricted diet does not help treat viral gastroenteritis.

Here are main tips you need to know about Norovirus, How do I prevent my family from getting sick? What is the difference between norovirus and rotavirus? Is it mostly affected by children or adult? What are transmission method? What are the treatment for it? The majority of norovirus outbreaks are caused by the GII.4 genotype, which has been the predominant circulating virus since 1995.

Chapter 1

What is the origin of Norovirus

Norovirus, an RNA virus of the family Caliciviridae, is a human gastrointestinal disease that causes high morbidity across both health care and community settings. Several factors improve the transmissibility of norovirus, including the minimal inoculum necessary to establish infection (<100 viral particles), persistent viral shedding, and its capacity

1

to survive in the environment. In this review, we explain the fundamental virology and immunology of noroviruses, the clinical illness arising from infection and its diagnosis and treatment, as well as host and pathogen characteristics that hamper vaccine development. Additionally, we examine general epidemiology, infection control techniques, and global reporting initiatives targeted at reducing this widespread source of acute gastroenteritis. Prompt deployment of infection control measures is the cornerstone of norovirus epidemic management.

Human norovirus, formerly known as Norwalk

2

virus, was initially detected in stool specimens collected during an epidemic of gastroenteritis in Norwalk, OH, and was the first viral agent demonstrated to cause gastroenteritis (1). (1). Illness attributable to this virus was originally identified in 1929 as "winter vomiting disease" because to its seasonal inclination and the frequent majority of patients with vomiting as a prominent symptom (2). (2).

The 1968 epidemic that led to the discovery of the virus afflicted 50% of pupils at an elementary school

3

 in Norwalk and manifested mostly as nausea, vomiting, diarrhea, and low-grade fever (3). (3). Among primary cases, 98% complained of nausea, and 92% vomited, while 58% experienced stomach cramps, 52% complained of fatigue, 38% had diarrhea, and 34% had fever. The incidence of secondary cases in 32% of family connections permitted the assumption of a 48-h incubation period. The sickness lasted ~24 h, with full recovery in all patients.

While no virus could be identified in the Norwalk epidemic, oral administration of filtrates made from

4

 rectal swabs from afflicted persons to healthy adult male convicts at the Maryland House of Correction in Jessup, MD, resulted in symptoms in 2 of 3 subjects (4). (4). In the 2 patients that fell sick, the incubation period was 48 h, as was the duration of symptoms. Mild diarrhea, with 4 to 6 loose stools, lasted 24 h, whereas low-grade fever lasted just 8 to 12 h. Other symptoms included anorexia, somewhat severe stomach cramps, malaise, headache, and nausea (but no vomiting) (but no vomiting). A full restoration to health happened within 96 h. The filtrate of a stool sample from 1 of the 2

5

symptomatic experimentally infected volunteers was subsequently fed to a further 9 participants, 7 of whom fell unwell. Two of the seven participants vomited (one person, who vomited ~20 times in 24 h, needed parenteral fluid replacement) but failed to develop diarrhea, whereas two had diarrhea without vomiting, and three had both diarrhea and vomiting. Four of the seven

participants experienced low-grade
fever that lasted 8 to 12 h, while all
seven subjects complained of malaise
and headache. Symptoms resolved
after a mean length of 33 h.

6

While the index epidemic and the
human volunteer studies that
followed offered an accurate picture
of the symptoms of norovirus

infection in previously healthy children and adults at a time when the etiologic agent was unknown, it was an incomplete one. Further findings, mentioned later in this study, have offered a more complicated and nuanced perspective of the illness. Human noroviruses are the major cause of epidemic gastroenteritis in all age categories and have been connected with high-profile outbreaks in hospitals, nursing homes, cruise ships, and the military (5, 6). (5, 6). It is estimated

7

that each year, noroviruses are responsible for 64,000 diarrheal episodes requiring hospitalization, 900,000 clinic visits among children in affluent countries, and ~200,000 fatalities of children <5 years old in the poor world.

Chapter 2

Symptoms of norovirus

The most frequent symptoms of norovirus are:

diarrhea

vomiting

nausea

9

stomach discomfort

Other symptoms include:

fever

headache

body aches

Do you believe you have the stomach flu or a stomach bug?

10

It is probably norovirus, a common virus that is not connected to the flu. Norovirus is the most prevalent cause of vomiting and diarrhea, and foodborne sickness.

Norovirus causes inflammation of the stomach or intestines. This is termed acute gastroenteritis.

A person generally develops symptoms 12 to 48 hours after being exposed to norovirus. Most persons with norovirus disease recover well within 1 to 3 days.

11

If you have norovirus infection, you might feel really unwell

Stomach Flu (Gastroenteritis) (Gastroenteritis)

Gastroenteritis is frequently dubbed "stomach flu." But it's really not caused by influenza, the respiratory virus that causes flu. Different stomach bugs (germs) are typically to responsible for symptoms including diarrhea, stomach discomfort and feeling ill to your stomach.

What is stomach flu (gastroenteritis)? Gastroenteritis is inflammation (irritation) of your intestines. People commonly term it a "stomach

12

bug" or "stomach flu," even though it's not restricted to just influenza. Although most patients experience stomach discomfort, gastroenteritis may also impact your small intestines and colon.

How often is stomach flu (gastroenteritis)?

Stomach flu is prevalent. More than 20 million individuals fall sick each year in the U.S. with a digestive disturbance. Viruses are the most prevalent cause of stomach flu.

Who gets stomach flu (gastroenteritis)?

13

Anyone may come sick with stomach flu. But you're more likely to acquire it if you're in a location where lots of people share living or eating areas, such as:

Children at childcare or at camp.

Nursing homes.

Students living in dorms.

Military troops.

Prisons.

Psychiatric wards.

Cruise-ship passengers.

Travelers visiting less-developed nations.

14

Anyone having immunological weakened status.

What causes stomach flu
(gastroenteritis)?

You may become ill from germs,
parasites, poisons and viruses.
Viruses are the most prevalent cause
of so-called stomach flu. Norovirus is
commonly the cause for adults,
while rotavirus is usually to blame
for stomach flu in youngsters. These
viruses mainly attack the lining of the
small intestine.

What are the symptoms of stomach flu (gastroenteritis)?

15

The major symptom of gastroenteritis is diarrhea. When the GI tract gets infected during gastroenteritis, numerous actions from the virus leads on diarrhea. Malabsorption occurs due of the breakdown of the intestinal cells called enterocytes.

The virus may also impair the reasbsorption of water and create secretory diarrhea, which is responsible for the loose liquidy stools.

Abdominal (belly) pain or cramping.

Nausea and vomiting.

Fever.

Headache and body pains.

16

Can stomach flu produce a fever?

You could acquire a fever when you have stomach flu. A fever might be an indication that your body is battling an illness. You may feel hot, clammy or have the chills. You may also feel a headache or soreness all throughout your body.

Is the stomach flu worse in certain people?

In general, most individuals recover quickly from the stomach flu.

Symptoms may be severe in newborns, young children, elderly people or anybody of any age who is immune-compromised. Vomiting and diarrhea may cause dehydration (not

18

 enough water in the body) within only a short amount of time, depending on the conditions. Signs of dehydration include:

Extreme thirst.

Less urine flow than normal (no wet diapers for three hours or more in newborns) (no wet diapers for three hours or more in infants).

Urine that is darker in hue.

Sunken cheeks or eyes.

Lightheadedness, dizziness upon standing.

General weakness.

Why does stomach flu attack at night?

19

In some persons, the stomach flu symptoms may be more prominent at night owing to their circadian cycle. At night an increase in immune system activity produces infection-fighting chemicals. These may trigger inflammation that make you feel worse while you combat your illness.

Is stomach flu (gastroenteritis) contagious?

Viral stomach flu spreads quickly to others. You may get a stomach flu virus any time of the year, but the common norovirus is more frequent from November to April when people tend to spend more

20

inside. Because a number of viruses may cause stomach flu, you could

have various kinds of gastroenteritis
numerous times during life.

It's passed from person to person by
getting into touch with small,
invisible particles from a sick
person's feces or vomit if you:
Touch a surface and come in contact
with the germs and you touch food or
your mouth.

Eat or consume food or drinks that
contain a sick person's germs.

21

Have close contact with someone who has stomach flu (even if they have no symptoms) (even if they have no symptoms).

When should you consult a doctor for stomach flu (gastroenteritis)?

You'll likely be able to fight off stomach flu virus without visiting a healthcare practitioner. If you experience indicators of dehydration (dark, infrequent/low urine production, dry mucous membranes, lightheadedness, dizziness, etc.), you should seek medical assistance straight once. Also notify your healthcare practitioner if you have:

22

High fever.

Bloody diarrhea.

Severe pain.

Symptoms that fail to

improve/resolve with time.

Chapter3

Ways of Transmission of Norovirus

Norovirus spreads extremely rapidly and swiftly in many ways. You may catch norovirus by accidently putting microscopic particles of feces (poop) or vomit from an infected individual in your mouth.

This may happen if you

24

consume food or drink drinks that are infected with norovirus,

contact surfaces or items infected
with norovirus and then put your
fingers in your mouth, or
having direct contact with someone
who is infected with norovirus, such
as by caring for them or sharing food
or eating utensils with them.

If you acquire norovirus infection,
you may shed billions of norovirus
particles that you couldn't detect
without a microscope. Only a few

norovirus particles may get other individuals ill. You are most contagious

25

when you have symptoms of norovirus disease, notably vomiting, and

over the first several days after you recover from norovirus sickness.

However, studies have shown that you may continue transmit norovirus for two weeks or more after you feel well.

Norovirus spreads via contaminated food

Norovirus may readily contaminate food and water since it just needs a very little quantity of virus particles to get you ill. Food and water may acquire contaminated with norovirus in several ways,

26

including when:

An infected person touches food with their bare hands that have feces (poop) or vomit particles on them

Food is placed on a counter or surface that has feces or vomit particles on it

Tiny drops of vomit from an infected person spray through the air and land on the food

The food is grown or harvested with contaminated water, such as oysters harvested from contaminated water, or fruit and vegetables irrigated with contaminated water in the field

27

Norovirus and Food

Norovirus is the leading cause of illness and outbreaks from contaminated food in the United States. Most of these outbreaks occur in food service environments like restaurants. Infected food workers are commonly the cause of outbreaks, typically by handling ready-to-eat goods, such as fresh fruits and vegetables, with their bare hands before serving them. However, any meal served uncooked or touched after being cooked might become infected with norovirus.

More

28

Norovirus spreads via polluted water

Recreational or drinking water may

be contaminated with norovirus and

make you ill or taint your meals. This

may happen:

At the source such as when a septic

tank overflows into a well

When an infected person vomits or

poops in the water

When water isn't treated properly,

such as with not enough chlorine

For more information on safe water

and how water may become polluted,

check

29

Norovirus spreads via ill persons and

contaminated surfaces

Surfaces may acquire contaminated

with norovirus in several ways,

including when:

An infected individual contacts the surface with their bare hands that have feces or vomit particles on them

An infected person vomits or has diarrhea that splatters onto surfaces

Food, water, or objects that are contaminated with norovirus are placed on surfaces

30

Tiny particles of vomit spray through the air and land on surfaces or enter a person's mouth, then he or she swallows it

Noroviruses are positive-sense, non-enveloped RNA viruses, which are a leading cause of viral gastroenteritis and a common cause of outbreaks in institutional settings. Infections with these viruses are difficult to prevent and control, as their genome recombines or mutates readily, and new variants can emerge every few years to become the dominant strains in a certain period.

31

The majority of norovirus outbreaks are caused by the GII.4 genotype, which has been the predominant circulating virus since 1995. The development of molecular-based diagnostic methods has provided better insight into the epidemiological impact of noroviruses, which is important to identify trends for the detection, prevention, and control of the disease.

Transmission routes

Several methods of norovirus transmission have been found owing to a plethora of well-documented outbreaks. In general, the person-to-person

32

 dissemination constitutes the predominant mechanism of transmission in epidemics. This remains true for endemic instances of norovirus infection, which are largely assisted by the low infectious dosage of between 18 and 1000 virus particles.

However, foodborne transmission may also play a crucial role, generally as a consequence of contamination by an infected food handler, which underlines the fecal-oral mode of transmission. In addition, some waterborne outbreaks have been

33

documented, and there is indirect evidence of possible airborne transmission, such as in explosive vomiting that occurred throughout the sickness.

In most situations, several mechanisms of transmission are responsible for epidemics. One example is when a food handler gets sick by person-to-person transmission at his or her home, and then subsequently contaminates a food product, resulting to a common cause epidemic. This, in turn, may proceed further via person-to-person transmission or environmental contamination.

Epidemiology of norovirus

34

Compilation of the top interviews, articles, and news in the recent year.

It is believed that roughly 200,000

people die each year from norovirus

infections, primarily in the

underdeveloped nations. Outbreaks

threaten health care institutions

globally, having the potential to

create a huge disruption in their

capacity to deliver treatment, severe

economic loss, and death among

susceptible patient populations.

Humans are assumed to be the sole host for human noroviruses, however recent identification of similar

35

noroviruses in pooled stool samples from calves and pigs has hinted at the potential of zoonotic transmission. As interspecies transmission has been confirmed for several animal caliciviruses, which are recognized for their extensive host range, animals as a possible reservoir for human infections remains a serious public health concern.

Norovirus excretion patterns may play an essential impact in the dissemination of the virus. Virion excretion may occur after all the primary symptoms have vanished, although norovirus RNA excretion can happen even before the beginning of symptoms.

36

Furthermore, the excretion might persist for lengthy periods of time, particularly in immunocompromised persons.

Chapter4

Norovirus

Prevention

You may help protect yourself and others from norovirus by washing your hands thoroughly with soap and water and following other basic preventative recommendations.

Practice good hand hygiene

Wash your hands thoroughly with soap and water

After using the restroom or changing diapers.

Before consuming, preparing, or
handling food.

38

Before giving yourself or someone
else medication.

Norovirus may be identified in your
vomit or feces (poop) even before
you start feeling unwell. The virus
may also persist in your feces for two
weeks or more after you feel well. It
is crucial to maintain washing your

hands regularly throughout this period.

Hand sanitizer does not function effectively against norovirus. Handwashing is always preferable. Wash your hands with soap and water for at least 20 seconds. You may use hand sanitizers in addition to hand washing, but hand sanitizer is not a replacement for washing

39

your hands with warm water and soap.

Handle and prepare food safely

Before preparing and consuming your food:

Carefully wash fruits and vegetables.

Cook oysters and other shellfish thoroughly to an internal temperature of at least 145°F .

Be mindful that noroviruses are relatively resistant to heat. They can endure temperatures as high as 145°F. Quick steaming techniques that are typically used for preparing shellfish may not heat foods sufficiently to destroy noroviruses.

40

Food that could be infected with norovirus should be thrown aside. People who are unwell should not prepare or handle food.

Clean and disinfect surfaces

After someone vomits or has

diarrhea, always thoroughly clean

and disinfect the whole area

immediately:

Put on rubber or disposable gloves

and wipe the whole area with paper

towels, then disinfect the area with a

bleach-based home cleaner as

instructed on the product label.

41

Leave the bleach disinfectant on the damaged area for at least five minutes, then rinse the whole area again with soap and hot water. Finish by cleaning dirty clothing, putting out the trash, and washing your hands.

To help make sure that food is safe from norovirus, frequently clean and sterilize kitchen equipment, worktops, and surfaces before

making meals.

You should use a chlorine bleach

solution with a concentration of

1,000 to 5,000 ppm (5 to 25

teaspoons of home bleach [5% to

8%] per gallon of

42

 water) or other disinfectant

designated as effective against

norovirus by the Environmental Protection Agency (EPA) (EPA).

Wash laundry thoroughly

Immediately remove and wash garments or linens that may be soiled with vomit or feces.

You should:

Handle filthy goods gently without disturbing (shaking) them.

Wear rubber or disposable gloves when handling filthy goods and wash your hands afterwards.

43

Wash the articles using detergent (cleaning agent) and hot water at the longest allowable cycle duration and then machine dry them at the highest heat setting.

5 Simple Tips to Prevent Norovirus This Winter

It's not only on cruise ships.

Norovirus – the most frequent cause of gastroenteritis, or "stomach flu" — is everywhere. And it's frequently tough to prevent.

The Centers for Disease Control and Prevention estimate that 1 in 15 U.S. citizens becomes ill with norovirus every year. Common symptoms include nausea, vomiting, diarrhea, abdominal pain and, on

44

sometimes, a low-grade fever. "People come into touch with norovirus via contaminated foods, contaminated water and sick persons who are preparing and handling food, as well as through person-to-person spread," says Camille Sabella, MD, Director of the Center for Pediatric

Infectious Diseases. It's widespread

in locations such as restaurants,

cruise ships and schools, but also in

day care facilities, nursing homes and

other public areas.

Norovirus normally peaks between

the months of December and April.

"That's very likely related to

45

people being closer together, where there's an opportunity for person-to-person contact," Dr. Sabella says.

It's extremely infectious, but there are methods to keep yourself and your family healthy this winter.

1. Wash your hands

It sounds easy because it is. Frequent hand-washing is arguably the best approach to avoid norovirus. Work up a nice lather with soap, then wash for at least 20 seconds.

Avoid contact with somebody who's recently had vomiting or diarrhea if you can. If you're exposed to

46

a sick individual, wash your hands quickly. If you are caring for someone with norovirus, wash your hands every time you come into touch with them. Hand sanitizer also may aid as an addition to hand-washing but not as an alternative.

2. Keep your hands away from your face

To catch this virus, you essentially have to consume it. That implies you should intentionally avoid touching your face. If you've touched anything that's infected with the virus, touching your mouth, nose or eyes before you have a chance to wash your hands makes it simpler for the

virus to enter your

47

 body.

3. Pay attention to your surroundings

You don't have to be a food

inspector to spot bad safety practices.

If you're getting takeout from a

restaurant where the food is not being

handled appropriately — for

instance, if people are directly

touching the food without gloves —

then find another place to eat.

4. Practice food safety at home

Remember tip No. 1 about hand-

washing? It is particularly critical in

the kitchen since norovirus spreads

via eating. As you prepare food,

wash your

48

hands frequently — especially right

before serving anything to others.

Also, if you have symptoms or know you are ill, keep out of the kitchen to prevent spreading the infection to others.

5. Use appropriate cleaning methods It might take several days for someone who is infected with norovirus to develop symptoms, Dr. Sabella notes. That means you can't always keep it out of your house —

and norovirus is difficult to contain
once it has entered your house.
Still, you can take steps to clean
up and prevent its spread. For
example, focus on scrubbing any

49

commonly touched surfaces such as
doorknobs and counter tops. Just
remember — the main sources of
transmission are contaminated foods
and person-to-person contact. That

means wiping a doorknob isn't going to be as effective as your absolute best prevention tip: Wash your hands.

Norovirus can't be treated with antibiotics, so if you catch it, simply wait it out and rest. "Drink plenty of water to avoid dehydration, wash your hands frequently and avoid contact with others to keep the virus from spreading,"

50

Chapter 5

Treatment

there is no particular treatment to treat persons with norovirus disease.

If you have norovirus disease, you should consume lots of liquids to replenish fluid lost through vomiting

and diarrhea. This will assist avoid

dehydration.

Dehydration may lead to major

issues. Severe

51

dehydration may necessitate

hospitalization for treatment with

fluids administered via your vein

(intravenous or IV fluids)

(intravenous or IV fluids).

Watch for indicators of dehydration

in children who have norovirus

sickness. Children who are

dehydrated may weep with little or

no tears and be particularly drowsy

or cranky.

If you suspect you or someone you

are caring for is very dehydrated,

contact your healthcare practitioner.

Drink lots of drinks to replenish

fluids that are lost through vomiting

and diarrhea. Sports drinks and

52

 other liquids without caffeine or

alcohol may assist with minor

dehydration. However, these

beverages may not replace key

nutrients and minerals. Oral

rehydration fluids that you may

obtain over the counter are most

useful for moderate dehydration.

Seasonal influenza is an acute

respiratory illness caused by

influenza viruses which circulate in

all regions of the globe.

It reflects a year-round illness load. It

causes symptoms that vary in

severity and can lead to

hospitalization and death.

53

Most individuals recover from fever and other symptoms within a week without needing medical intervention. However, influenza may cause severe illness or death, especially among high risk populations including the very young, the elderly, pregnant women, health professionals and individuals with chronic medical problems.

In temperate areas, seasonal epidemics occur largely during winter, whereas in tropical places, influenza may exist throughout the year, generating outbreaks more sporadically.

54

Chapter 6

Treatment of Viral Gastroenteritis ("Stomach Flu")

How can I cure viral gastroenteritis?

In most situations, persons with viral

gastroenteritis get well on their own

without medical treatment. You can

treat viral gastroenteritis by restoring

lost

55

 fluids and electrolytes to

prevent dehydration. In certain

circumstances, over-the-counter

drugs may help ease your symptoms.

Research demonstrates that

maintaining a limited diet does not

help cure viral gastroenteritis. When you have viral gastroenteritis, you may vomit after you eat or lose your appetite for a brief period. When your hunger returns, you can most likely go back to eating your usual diet, even if you still have diarrhea. Find recommendations on what to eat when you have viral gastroenteritis.

56

If your kid develops signs of viral gastroenteritis, such as vomiting or diarrhea, don't hesitate to contact a doctor for help.

Replace lost fluids and electrolytes

When you have viral gastroenteritis, you need to restore lost fluids and electrolytes to avoid dehydration or cure moderate dehydration. You should drink lots of liquids. If vomiting is a concern, try swallowing

little quantities of clear drinks.

57

Most individuals with viral

gastroenteritis may replenish fluids

and electrolytes with beverages such

as

water

fruit juices

sports drinks

broths

Eating saltine crackers may also help

restore electrolytes.

If your child has viral gastroenteritis,

you should give your kid an oral

rehydration solution—

58

such as Pedialyte, Naturalyte,

Infalyte, and CeraLyte—as instructed

to replenish lost fluids and electrolytes. Oral rehydration solutions are liquids that contain glucose and electrolytes. Talk with a doctor before administering these remedies to your newborn. Infants should swallow breast milk or formula as normal. Older individuals, adults with a weakened immune system, and adults with severe diarrhea or indications of dehydration should additionally take oral rehydration solutions.

59

Over-the-counter medications

In rare circumstances, adults may use over-the-counter drugs such as loperamide NIH external link (Imodium) and bismuth subsalicylate NIH external

link (Pepto-Bismol, Kaopectate) to

treat diarrhea caused by viral

gastroenteritis.

These drugs might be harmful for

newborns and toddlers. Talk with a

doctor before giving your kid an

over-the-counter drug.

If you have bloody diarrhea or

fever—signs of infections

with bacteria or parasites—don't use

over

60

the-counter drugs to treat diarrhea.

See a doctor for treatment.

How do doctors treat viral

gastroenteritis?

Your doctor may prescribe drugs to

manage extreme vomiting. Doctors

don't prescribe antibiotics NIH

external link to treat viral

gastroenteritis. Antibiotics don't work for viral infections.

In certain situations, your doctor may recommend probiotics NIH external link. Probiotics are living microorganisms, most typically bacteria, that are like the ones you naturally have in your digestive system. Studies show that certain

61

probiotics may help shorten an

episode of diarrhea. Researchers are

still exploring the effectiveness of

probiotics to treat viral

gastroenteritis. For safety concerns,

speak with your doctor before taking

probiotics or any

other complementary or alternative

medications or practices NIH

external link.

Anyone with signs or symptoms of dehydration should visit a doctor straight once. Doctors may need to treat persons with severe dehydration in a hospital.

How can I avoid viral gastroenteritis?

62

You may take many actions to avoid from having or spreading viruses that cause viral gastroenteritis. Wash your

hands thoroughly with soap and

water

after using the bathroom

after changing diapers

before and after touching, preparing,

or ingesting food

You may clean objects that may have

come into touch with infected feces

or vomit, including as worktops and

changing tables, using a combination

of 5 to 25 teaspoons of household

bleach and

63

1 gallon of water.

If clothing or linens may have come

into touch with an infected person's

feces or vomit, you should wash

them with detergent on the longest

cycle possible and machine dry them.

To protect yourself from illness, use

rubber gloves when handling the dirty clothing and wash your hands afterward.

If you have viral gastroenteritis, avoid handling and preparing food for others while you are unwell and for 2 days after your symptoms cease.

People who have viral gastroenteritis may transfer the infection to any meal they touch, particularly if they do not completely wash their hands. Contaminated water may potentially transfer a virus to foods before they are harvested. For example, infected fruits, vegetables, and oysters have been connected to norovirus outbreaks. Wash fruits and vegetables before using them, and fully cook oysters and other shellfish.

Find ideas to help keep food safe External link.

65

The flu vaccine NIH external link does not protect against viral gastroenteritis. Although some individuals term viral gastroenteritis "stomach flu," influenza (flu) viruses NIH external link do not cause viral gastroenteritis. However, rotavirus vaccines can prevent viral gastroenteritis caused by rotavirus.

Rotavirus Vaccines

Two vaccines, which infants receive by mouth, are approved to protect against rotavirus infections

RotaTeq: Infants receive three doses, at ages 2 months, 4 months, and 6 months

Rotarix: Infants receive this vaccine in two doses, at ages 2 months and 4 months

For the rotavirus vaccination to be most effective, newborns should get the first dose by 15 weeks of age. Infants should get all doses by 8 months of age.

If you have a baby, consult with your baby's doctor about rotavirus vaccination External link.

This information is provided as a service of the National Institute of Diabetes and Digestive and

67

Kidney Diseases (NIDDK), part of the National Institutes of Health. The NIDDK interprets and disseminates research results to expand knowledge and understanding about health and illness among patients, health professionals, and the public. Content provided by the NIDDK is thoroughly vetted by NIDDK scientists and other professionals.

What is the difference between norovirus and the stomach flu? Norovirus causes gastroenteritis, which some people may term the "stomach flu." The influenza virus causes respiratory flu, not

gastroenteritis.

68

Chapter 7

How many Types of

norovirus exist?

There are various distinct varieties (strains) of norovirus. It's in the Caliciviridae family of viruses that cause inflammation of your stomach and intestines (gastroenteritis) (gastroenteritis). In this family, there are 10 groups with 48 types. The most prevalent kind is GII.4.

69

How prevalent is norovirus?

Norovirus is quite prevalent.

Globally, roughly 685 million cases

are recorded each year. Of that

estimate, nearly 200 million

instances harm children.

Is norovirus seasonal?

Norovirus outbreaks occur most

commonly between November and

April in countries above the equator

and between April and September in

countries below the equator. There's

generally no distinct season for epidemics in locations on the equator.

Are norovirus symptoms the same in children and adults?

70

Symptoms of norovirus are typically the same in both children and adults. Adults may have more diarrhea than children and toddlers may vomit more than adults.

What are the risk factors for norovirus?

Anyone may acquire norovirus.

You're more likely to develop norovirus,

You come into touch with someone who has the virus.

Your genes make you more prone to have symptoms (genetic susceptibility) (genetic susceptibility).

What are the problems of norovirus?

71

If you have norovirus, you'll feel really unwell. This might cause you to vomit up and have diarrhea. When you're unable to store nutrients in your body, you're at danger of dehydration. Symptoms of dehydration include:

Peeing less frequently or having dark-colored urine.

Having a dry mouth.

Feeling weak or dizzy.

A headache.

Children may experience the

aforementioned symptoms, along

with:

Crying without tears.

72

Fussiness.

Sleepiness throughout the day.

Norovirus might make it difficult for you to eat or drink because the inflammation in your intestines and stomach leads you to vomit or have diarrhea. You still need to make an effort to eat and drink. You can do this by eating and drinking more often throughout the day, eating slowly and taking small bites or taking little sips of fluids. If you eat too rapidly or too much, your body may reject the food intake.

73

Can norovirus be prevented?

Some actions you may take to lower your chance of having norovirus include:

Washing your hands regularly with soap and water.

Washing your food before consuming it (fruits and veggies) (fruits and vegetables).

Cooking your meal thoroughly (particularly seafood or shellfish) or to a suitable temperature (at least 145 degrees Fahrenheit, or 62.77 degrees Celsius) (at least 145 degrees Fahrenheit, or 62.77 degrees Celsius).

Avoiding contact with those who have a norovirus infection.

Cleaning and sanitizing regularly touched surfaces and items.

Washing your garments thoroughly, particularly if they're filthy.

Using hand sanitizer doesn't destroy norovirus particles as efficiently as washing your hands with soap and warm water. If you have a norovirus illness, you shouldn't make meals or take care of others, since you're at danger of transmitting the sickness. 75

Chapter 8

Can you catch norovirus twice?

Yes, you can get norovirus more than once. There are various forms of noroviruses. Your body may establish a little immunity (protection from the virus) against the first kind of norovirus, but not other varieties. This implies you may become ill with norovirus several times during your life. If you

76

do have an immunity to a form of norovirus, it may not stay forever.

This implies that there might be a considerable gap of time between your first and second illnesses.

What can I anticipate if I have norovirus?

Norovirus symptoms are frequently abrupt and unpleasant. You'll likely be throwing up (vomiting) or experiencing diarrhea for a few days until the illness takes its course. The notion of eating or drinking might be repulsive. But you'll put yourself at danger of dehydration if you don't eat or drink. If you're unable to eat or drink, consult a healthcare

77

practitioner.

There are various strains of norovirus, so if you get ill once, it's possible you may become sick again, since your body hasn't established an immune to every form of norovirus.

The disease is transient and doesn't generally produce any long-term damage.

How long does norovirus remain in my system?

When norovirus enters your body, it's present in your stool (poop) before you have symptoms. It may also linger in your system for up to two weeks after your symptoms go gone. You're only infectious when you get sick until 48 hours after your

78

 symptoms end.

When should I visit a healthcare provider?

Visit a healthcare practitioner if you're unable to eat or drink. This may lead to dehydration. You should also contact your provider if you experience symptoms that extend longer than three days.

What questions should I ask my doctor?

Do I have norovirus or another form of infection?

How do I eat or drink while I'm sick?

Can I take any drugs to help me feel better?

How can I protect my family from becoming sick?

79

Chapter 9

What is the difference between norovirus and rotavirus?

Both norovirus and rotavirus are infections that cause inflammation of your stomach and intestines (gastroenteritis), but they're separate illnesses.

Norovirus

1 Caused by a strain of Caliciviridae.

80

2 Infection lasts between one and three days.

3 Affects anybody at any age.

4There isn't a vaccination available.

Rotavirus

1 Caused by a strain of Reoviridae.

2 Infection lasts between three

and\seight days.

3 Affects usually youngsters

and\ssometimes adults.

4 There's a vaccination available.

A message from Cleveland Clinic

Norovirus is a sudden and frustrating sickness. You need to eat and drink, yet your body has difficulties

81

keeping it down. Luckily, the condition only lasts for a few days. You might attempt to eat and drink little nibbles or sips periodically throughout the day instead of eating huge meals. Contact your healthcare physician if you can't eat or if your symptoms continue longer than three days. Make sure you wash your hands regularly with soap and water to avoid the spread of the illness.

82